Published By Adam Gilbin

@ Luther Reyes

Belly Fat: Simple Guides on How to Burn Bad Fat

and Archiving a Flat Stomach and Fitness

ISBN 978-1-990666-75-9

I0554684

TABLE OF CONTENTS

Italian Vegetable Soup

Ingredients:

- few sprigs thyme

- 3 courgettes, chopped

- 400g can butter beans, drained

- 400g can chopped tomatoes

- 1.2l vegetable stock

- 100g parmesan or vegetarian equivalent, grated

- 140g small pasta shapes

- small bunch basil, shredded

- 2 each of onions and carrots, chopped

- 4 sticks celery, chopped

- 1 tbsp olive oil

- 2 tbsp sugar

- 4 garlic cloves, crushed

- 2 tbsp tomato purée

- 2 bay leaves

Directions:

1. Gently cook the onion, carrots and celery in the oil in a large saucepan for 20 mins, until soft. Splash in water if they stick.

2. Add the sugar, garlic, purée, herbs and courgettes and cook for 4-5 mins on a medium heat until they brown a little.

3. Pour in the beans, tomatoes and stock, then simmer for 20 mins. If you're freezing it, cool and do so now (freeze for up to three months). If not, add half the Parmesan and the pasta and simmer for 6-8 mins until pasta cooked.

4. Sprinkle with basil and remaining Parmesan to serve. If frozen, defrost then re-heat before

adding pasta and cheese and continuing as
above.

Red Pepper-Scallion Corn Muffin

Ingredients:

- 1/4 tsp baking soda

- 1/8 tsp freshly ground black pepper

- 1 c fat-free plain yogurt

- 1 large egg

- 2 large egg whites

- 2 tsp brown sugar

- 3/4 c drained canned vacuum-packed corn kernels (about 1/2 an 11-ounce can)

- 2 Tbsp + 1/4 c canola oil, divided

- 1 large red bell pepper, coarsely chopped

- 4 scallions, thinly sliced

- 1½ c yellow cornmeal

- 1/2 c whole grain pastry flour

- 1¾ tsp baking powder

- 1/2 tsp salt

Directions:

1. Preheat oven to 350°F. Coat Texas-size, 6-cup muffin tin with cooking spray or line with paper baking cups.

2. Warm 2 Tbsp of the oil in medium skillet over medium heat.

3. Add bell pepper and cook, stirring, 5 minutes or until tender.

4. Add scallions. Cook, stirring, 1 minute or until softened. Remove from heat and let cool 5 minutes.

5. Stir together cornmeal, flour, baking powder, salt, baking soda, and black pepper in large bowl. In medium bowl, whisk together yogurt, egg, egg whites, sugar, and remaining 1/4 c oil. Fold in bell pepper mixture and corn.

6. Fold into dry INGREDIENTS: until just moistened.

7. Divide batter evenly among prepared muffin cups. Bake 25 to 30 minutes or until wooden pick inserted in center comes out clean.

8. Cool in pan on wire rack 5 minutes. Remove muffins from pan to cool completely on wire rack.

Hearty Roast Beef Panini

Ingredients:

- 1/4 avocado, sliced

- 1/8 cup baby arugula

- 1 tsp Dijon mustard

- 1/4 tsp extra virgin olive oil

- 2 slices reduced-calorie multigrain bread

- 2 ounces store-roasted, deli-sliced lean roast beef

- 2 beefsteak tomato slices

Directions:

1. Place 1 slice of the bread on a work surface.
2. Top with the roast beef, tomato slices, avocado slices, and arugula.
3. Spread the remaining bread with mustard and set, mustard side down, on the arugula.

4. Heat a ridged nonstick grill pan over medium heat until hot.

5. Lightly brush the outsides of the sandwich with the oil and place on the pan.

6. Set a heavy-bottomed skillet on top of the sandwich and cook for 1 to 2 minutes per side or until toasted and warm in the center.

A Nice Rice Pudding

Ingredients:

- 700ml semi-skimmed milk

- Pinch grated nutmeg

- 1 bay leaf , or strip lemon zest

- 100g pudding rice

- 50g sugar

Directions:

1. Heat oven to 150C/fan 130C/gas 2. Wash the rice and drain well. Butter an 850ml heatproof baking dish, then tip in the rice and sugar and stir through the milk. Sprinkle the nutmeg over and top with the bay leaf or lemon zest.

2. Cook for 2 hrs or until the pudding wobbles ever so slightly when shaken.

Grilled Cobb Salad

Ingredients:

- Freshly ground black pepper

- 1 bunch scallions

- 1 pint cherry tomatoes

- 1 avocado, cut into 1-inch pieces

- ½ cup mint leaves

- ¼ cup chopped toasted pistachios

- 1½ cups quinoa

- 1 tea spoon kosher salt, plus more

- 3 table spoons fresh lemon juice

- ¼ cup olive oil, plus more

- Flaky sea salt

Directions:

1. Bring quinoa, 1 tsp. kosher salt, and 3 cups water to a boil in a medium saucepan.

2. Cover, reduce heat to low, and simmer until quinoa is tender, 8–10 minutes.

3. Remove pan from heat and let sit 15 minutes.

4. Fluff quinoa with a fork; transfer to a large bowl.

5. Whisk lemon juice and ¼ cup oil in a small bowl.

6. Drizzle over warm quinoa and toss to coat; season with salt and pepper. Let cool.

7. Prepare a grill for medium-high heat.

8. Grill scallions and tomatoes in a grill basket, turning occasionally, until charred in spots and tomatoes begin to split, 6–8 minutes.

9. Transfer to a cutting board and slice scallions into 1" pieces.

10. Spoon quinoa onto a platter and top with scallions, tomatoes, avocado, mint, and pistachios.

11. Drizzle with oil and sprinkle with sea salt.

Quinoa Salad With Peaches And Pickled Onions

Ingredients:

- 3 Tbsp. sugar

- 2 large ripe firm peaches, cut into ½" pieces

- 1/2 bunch arugula, thick stems trimmed, leaves torn (about 2 cups)

- 2 cups small cherry tomatoes (about 1 pint), halved

- 1/4 cup olive oil

- 1/2 cup ½" pieces chives, divided

- 1 1/2 cups quinoa (any color) rinsed well

- 1 medium red onion, sliced ¼" thick

- 1/2 cup apple cider vinegar

- 4 tsp. kosher salt plus more

- Freshly ground black pepper

Directions:

1. Bring quinoa and 4 cups water to a boil in a medium saucepan. Season with salt.

2. Cover, reduce heat, and simmer until quinoa is tender, 8–10 minutes.

3. Drain, return quinoa to pan, and cover. Remove from heat and let sit 15 minutes.

4. Fluff with a fork and spread out on a rimmed baking sheet; let cool.

5. Meanwhile, place onion in a small bowl. Bring vinegar, sugar, and 4 tsp. salt to a boil in a small saucepan, stirring to dissolve sugar and salt.

6. Pour over onion and let stand 20 minutes. Drain, reserving pickling liquid.

7. Toss pickled onion, peaches, arugula, tomatoes, oil, ¼ cup chives, and 3 Tbsp. reserved pickling liquid in a large bowl; season with salt, pepper, and more pickling liquid, if desired. Fold in quinoa.

8. Serve salad topped with remaining ¼ cup chives.

Nutty Almond Pecan Cookies

Ingredients:

- 1/2 teaspoon sea salt

- 1 large egg yolk

- 3 tablespoons Grade B maple syrup

- 2 tablespoons extra-virgin olive oil

- 1 tablespoon unsweetened applesauce

- 2 cups (192 grams) blanched almond flour

- 1/2 cup raw pecans, finely chopped, plus about 30 pecan halves for garnish

- 3 tablespoons coconut sugar

- 1/2 teaspoon baking soda

Directions:

1. In a large bowl, whisk together the almond flour, chopped pecans, coconut sugar, baking soda, and salt. In a small bowl, whisk together

16

the egg yolk, maple syrup, olive oil, and applesauce.

2. Pour the wet INGREDIENTS: into the dry and stir to form dough.

3. Divide the dough in half. Roll each half into a log about 6 inches long and 1-1/2 to 2 inches in diameter. Wrap both logs in plastic wrap and freeze for 1-2 hours.

4. Preheat the oven to 350ºF. Line 2 baking sheets with parchment paper.

5. Slice the frozen dough logs into 1/4-inch thick rounds.

6. Place the cookies about 2 inches apart on the lined baking sheets.

7. Gently press a pecan half into the center of each cookie.

8. Bake for 12 to 15 minutes until golden brown and fragrant. Cool completely before serving. Store in an airtight container.

Dairy-Free Carrot Cake Ice Cream

Ingredients:

- 1/8 teaspoon salt

- 8 ounces Galaxy Classic Plain Vegan Cream Cheese Alternative

- 8 ounces plain dairy-free Greek yogurt (or regular dairy-free yogurt in a pinch)

- 2 cups 100% carrot juice

- 3/4 cup sugar

- 1 Tablespoon lemon juice

- 1/2 teaspoon vanilla extract

Directions:

1. Combine all INGREDIENTS: in a food processor or blender. Process or blend until smooth.
2. Chill in a glass container in the refrigerator for two hours.

3. Carefully pour into prepared ice cream maker and freeze according to its Directions:.

4. Eat as soft serve, or place in a glass container and freeze until firm.

5. Remove from freezer and let soften a few minutes before serving.

Banana-Raspberry With Coconut Milk And Sunflower Seeds

Ingredients:

- 1 cup fresh raspberries

- 1 tbsp sunflower seeds

- 1 pc large ripe banana, sliced

- ½ cup coconut milk

Directions:

1. In a bowl, place sliced banana and top with creamy coconut milk.
2. Add raspberries and sunflower seeds. Lightly toss. This makes 1 to 2 servings.

Quinoa-Orange Porridge

Ingredients:

- ½ cup water

- 1 pc fresh orange, peeled and chopped.

- 50g quinoa

- ½ cup rice milk

Directions:

1. Mix rice milk and water in saucepan set over low to medium fire.
2. Add quinoa and bring to a boil. Let it simmer until tender, or until all the liquid has been fully absorbed.
3. Remove from fire. Stir in chopped oranges and serve in a bowl. This makes 2-3 servings.

Mixed Berries With Yogurt And Pumpkin Seeds

Ingredients:

- 200g natural live yogurt (or Greek yogurt, or plain, unsweetened yogurt)

- 1 tbsp pumpkin seeds

- 200g berries (any type), fresh (if frozen or tinned, choose unsweetened ones)

Directions:

1. Place all INGREDIENTS: in a blender, and blend thoroughly.

2. To round up your breakfast, try adding a piece or slice of any fruit. You may also drink milk or add some cheese since they do not contain any wheat. Check the labels, though, since some types of cottage cheese may contain wheat fillers. Be careful of the type of milk, since there are flavored ones that contain wheat, such as malted milk.

3. If you are to add eggs to your breakfast, it would be better to consume them in the usual manners: scrambled, fried, or hard-boiled. If you try making quiche or soufflés, it is more than likely that you will have to use other INGREDIENTS: that contain wheat.

4. THIS IS IMPORTANT: when preparing meals, make sure that the INGREDIENTS: do not come into contact with other INGREDIENTS: that contain wheat. This is to prevent contamination. Therefore, see to it that you have separate tools or utensils for preparing regular meals (for those who are not following the wheat-free diet) and for preparing wheat-free meals.

Brown Rice Crust Quiche

INGREDIENTS:

For the brown rice crust

- 1 ½ cups of cooked brown rice

- 1 egg

For the filling

- 1 cup milk (you can likewise utilize a milk substitute, for example, almond milk)

- 4 eggs

- 2 cups of filling (you can look over changed kinds to be introduced below)

- ¼ teaspoon of salt

- ¼ teaspoon of pepper

Directions:

1. Preheat the stove to 350 degrees. Blend the rice in with the egg (1 egg).

2. Place the combination on a 9" tart or pie dish. Make certain to spread it equally, including the sides of the dish. You can either lube the dish ahead of time or not.

3. Bake the outside for around 10-15 minutes or until it becomes brilliant in shading. Set aside.

4. Whisk the elements for the filling together. Pour the blend onto the crust.

5. Bake it at 350 degrees for around 45 minutes, or until you see a toothpick tells the truth after you embed it at the center.

6. Let the quiche cool for around 10 minutes before you cut it up and serve.

7. You can decide to substitute the entire egg with egg whites. The various ideas for fillings incorporate the following:

8. Vegetarians: Chopped onions, spinach, tomatoes, and chime peppers Meat Lovers: Pepperoni, bacon, turkey, salami, ham Mediterranean: Roasted red peppers,

kalamata olives, tricks, artichoke hearts

Hawaiian: Onions, pineapple, Canadian bacon

Leftovers: Check your cooler for any extras
and pop them in your quiche.

Goat Cheese And Roast Tomatoes Stuffed Portobello Mushrooms

Ingredients:

- 2 tsp. shallot, finely cleaved (This is optional.)

- 1 tbsp. lemon juice

- 1 garlic clove (enormous), finely chopped

- 4 ounces goat cheddar (plain)

- 1 tbsp. new cleaved chives

- 1 tbsp. new cleaved parsley

- 4 Portobello mushrooms, around 4 inches across

- 3 tbsp. olive oil

- Oven cooked tomatoes

- Salt and pepper

Directions:

1. Clean the Portobello mushrooms by cleaning the external piece of the covers gently,using a moist paper towel, or forget about any soil utilizing a delicate brush.

2. Take out the stems by pushing them starting with one side then onto the next until they snap off. Utilizing a teaspoon, scratch the gills of the mushroom until the part under the mushroom is clean.

3. Place the mushrooms on rimmed baking sheet with a foil lining.

4. Mix lemon juice, garlic, shallot, and olive oil together. Brush the mushroom covers all around with the combination. You should then sprinkle each cap with pepper and salt.
   - Preheat the grill. Make certain to put the stove rack fair and square underneath the top level.

5. Broil the mushrooms for around 3 to 5 minutes until the edges begin to brown and the mushrooms become hot. Notice that they will become delicious and delivery moisture.

6. Remove mushrooms from the oven.

7. Preheat broiler to 375 degrees Fahrenheit. In the interim, fill the mushroom covers with simmered tomatoes and speck them with goat cheddar. Sprinkle them with new herbs.

8. Bake the mushrooms for 12 minutes or until the cheddar has mellowed. You can brush the edges of the covers with additional olive oil to make them shinier and serve.

Quick Fruit Smoothie

Ingredients:

- 3 peaches

- 3 cups of ice

- 2 cup of orange and mango juice

- 2 cup of strawberries

- 2 banana (cut in chunks)

Directions:

1. Add banana, strawberries, and peaches in a blender.
2. Blend until frothy and smooth.
3. Add the orange and mango juice and blend again.
4. Add ice for adjusting the consistency and blend for two minutes.
5. Divide the smoothie in glasses and serve with mango chunks from the top.

Triple Threat Smoothie

Ingredients:

- 2 kiwi (sliced)
- 2 banana (chopped)
- 2 cup of each
- Ice cubes
- Strawberries
- 1 cup of blueberries
- 2-4cup of orange juice
- 9 ounces of peach yogurt

Directions:

1. Add kiwi, strawberries, and bananas in a food processor.
2. Blend until smooth.
3. Add the blueberries along with orange juice. Blend again for two minutes.

4. Add peach yogurt and ice cubes. Give it a pulse.

5. Pour the prepared smoothie in smoothie glasses and serve with blueberry chunks from the top.

Fried Eggs And Bacon

Ingredients:

- 2 Eggs

- 3 Slices Bacon

Directions:

1. Heat the oil in your deep fryer to 375 degrees.
2. Cook the bacon in a pan and flip often until browned.
3. Crack the eggs in a dish and slowly slide them into the hot oil.
4. Corral the eggs into a ball and fry until it stops bubbling.
5. Drain in paper towels.

Ham And Egg Omelet

Ingredients:

- 12 Eggs

- 120 ml of Cream

- Salt, Pepper

- Onion Powder

- Garlic Powder to taste

- 1 Ham (3/4 lb.), diced

- 2 Bunches of Green Onions (12 Green onions), sliced

- 14.5 Oz Can Diced Tomatoes, drained

- 9 Slices Monterey Jack Cheese

Directions:

1. Preheat your oven to 350 degrees F.
2. Mix the cream, eggs, salt, onion powder and garlic powder.

3. Grease the muffin pan and fill it with the egg mixture.

4. Bake for 4-5 min.

5. Add the vegetables and bake for 7-8 min. or until set.

6. Sprinkle the cheese and bake for 1 min.

Low-Fat Whole-Wheat Pancakes

Ingredients:

- 2 cups whole-wheat flour

- 1 ½ tablespoons organic cane sugar

- 1 teaspoon baking powder

- ½ teaspoon baking soda

- 2 cups skim milk

- 2 tablespoons apple cider vinegar

- 5 egg whites, beaten well

- ¼ cup unsweetened applesauce

Directions:

1. Whisk together the milk and vinegar in a small bowl – let rest 5 minutes.

2. Combine the dry INGREDIENTS: in a mixing bowl and stir well.

3. In another bowl, beat the egg whites, applesauce, and milk mixture until smooth.

4. Whisk the wet INGREDIENTS: into the dry until well combined.

5. Heat a large skillet over medium-high heat and grease with cooking spray.

6. Spoon the batter into the pan using about 2 tablespoons per pancake.

7. Cook for 2 minutes or until bubbles form in the surface of the batter then flip and cook for 2 minutes more.

8. Slide the pancakes onto a plate and repeat with the remaining batter.

Strawberry Kale Green Smoothie

Ingredients:

- 1 cup skim milk

- ½ cup ice cubes

- 1 tablespoon ground flaxseed

- 2 cups fresh chopped kale

- ½ cup frozen sliced strawberries

- 1 ripe kiwi, peeled and sliced

Directions:

1. Combine all of the INGREDIENTS: in a high-speed blender.
2. Blend for 30 to 60 seconds on high speed until smooth.
3. Pour the smoothie into a glass and enjoy immediately.

Grape Smoothie

Ingredients:

- ¼ cup orange juice

- 1 cup unsweetened almond milk

- 3 ice cubes

- ½ cup blueberries

- ½ cup frozen red grapes

- 1 banana, peeled and frozen

- 1/8 teaspoon ground cinnamon

Directions:

1. Add all the INGREDIENTS: into a blender and process until smooth.

Oat Berry Smoothie

Ingredients:

- 3 tablespoons honey

- ½ cup frozen berries

- 1 cup milk

- ½ cup old fashioned rolled oats

- ¼ cup ice

- ½ cup vanilla yogurt

Directions:

1. Put all the INGREDIENTS: into your blender and process until smooth.
2. Taste and add more honey to sweeten it or you can add more milk to make it thicker.

Peach And Oat Smoothie

Ingredients:

- 5.3 oz. Greek yogurt

- 1 cup almond milk

- 1 ½ cups peeled and diced peaches

- ½ cup water

- ½ cup oats

- 1 ripe banana, peeled and frozen

Directions:

1. Put all the INGREDIENTS: in a blender and process until smooth and creamy.

Chicken Piccata

Ingredients:

- 2 Tbsp chopped fresh parsley

- 2 tsp capers, minced

- Freshly ground black pepper

- 12 ounces boneless, skinless chicken tenders

- 2 Tbsp flour

- 4 Tbsp olive oil

- 2 freshly squeezed lemon juice

Directions:

1. LAY the tenders on a work surface. With a smooth scaloppine pounder or a rolling pin covered in plastic wrap, flatten to 1/4" thickness. Dredge the cutlets lightly in the flour.

2. HEAT a large skillet over medium-high heat. Add the oil to the skillet and heat until sizzling. Place the chicken in the skillet. Cook for 2 minutes per side or until lightly browned and cooked through.

3. ADD the lemon juice, parsley, and capers. Bring the mixture to a boil. Reduce the heat and simmer for 2 minutes to allow the flavors to blend. Season to taste with the pepper. Serve the chicken with the pan juices.

4. Note: Pounding the chicken breasts to an even thickness is an important step because it allows the chicken to cook evenly so both ends are moist and delicious.

Full Green Bean Casserole

Ingredients:

- 16 ounces thawed green beans, French-cut

- 8 ounces cubed cream cheese

- 3 tablespoons Parmesan cheese, grated

- 1 cup chicken broth

- 1/8 teaspoon red pepper, ground

- 4 tablespoons coconut oil or butter, divided

- 1/4 cup ground flaxseed

- 1 large onion, yellow – chopped

- 1 large onion, yellow – cut into rings

- 4 ounces sliced button mushrooms

Directions:

1. Preheat oven to 350F. Grease a 2-quart baking dish.

2. Over medium heat in a large skillet, heat 2 of
    4 tablespoons of oil or butter.

3. Add your onion rings and cook them. Stir
    occasionally as they cook for about 10
    minutes, or until they are lightly browned.

4. Place flaxseeds on a plate. Add your browned
    onion rings and coat with flaxseed. Set them
    to the side.

5. Using the same skillet on medium-high heat,
    add the other 2 tablespoons of oil or butter
    and heat.

6. Cook mushrooms and chopped onion for eight
    minutes, until they absorb most of the liquid.

7. Add broth and green beans and heat to
    simmer. Stir in cream cheese until it melts.

8. Stir in red pepper and Parmesan cheese.

9. Pour mixture into your baking dish and
    arrange onion rings on top.

10. Bake the casserole for about 25 minutes, until
    it is bubbling and hot.

Onion Rings For A Green Bean Casserole

Ingredients:

- 1 egg

- 1 tablespoon melted olive or coconut oil

- 1/2 cup almond meal

- 1 cup ground flaxseed

- 3/4 cup divided coconut flour

- 1/2 teaspoon smoked paprika

- 2 sweet onions, large in size, separated in rings after being cut into 1/2 inch thick slices

Directions:

1. Preheat your oven to 450F. Spray cooking spray to coat two baking sheets.

2. Combine one quarter cup of paprika and coconut flour in a small bowl.

3. Using another bowl, beat the oil and egg until they are blended.

4. Use a large plate to combine the almond meal, 1/2 cup of coconut flour and the flaxseed.

5. Drench onion rings in the paprika-coconut flour mixture.

6. Shake off any extra mixture gently.

7. Dip the rings into the egg mixture, and allow the excess to drip off. Coat with the flaxseed mixture.

8. Place onion rings on baking sheets and coat lightly with the cooking spray.

9. Bake onion rings for 12 minutes or until browned. Turn them once while baking.

Easy Lentil Curry

Ingredients:

- 850ml vegetable stock

- 750g stewpack frozen vegetables

- 100g red lentil

- 200g basmati rice

- 2 tbsp sunflower oil

- 2 medium onions, cut into rough wedges

- 4 tbsp curry paste

- Turmeric

- Handful of raisins and roughly chopped parsley

- Poppadums and mango chutney, to serve

Directions:

1. Heat the oil in a large pan. Add the onions and cook over a high heat for about 8 minutes or until they are golden brown.

2. Stir in the curry paste and cook for a minute. Slowly pour in a little of the stock so it sizzles, scraping any bits from the bottom of the pan. Gradually pour in the rest of the stock.

3. Stir the frozen vegetables, cover and simmer for 5 minutes.

4. Add the lentils and simmer for a further 15-20 minutes or until the vegetables and lentils are cooked.

5. While the curry is simmering, cook the rice according to the packet instructions, adding the turmeric to the cooking water. Drain well.

6. Season the curry with salt, toss in a handful of raisins and chopped parsley, then serve with the rice, poppadums and chutney.

Jewelled Cranberry & Juniper Red Cabbage

Ingredients:

- 1 large red cabbage , shredded

- 300ml good-quality apple juice

- 300g fresh or frozen cranberries

- 2 tbsp light olive oil

- 2 onions , halved and thinly sliced

- 1 tsp juniper berries, lightly crushed

Directions:

1. Heat the oil in a large lidded pan, then gently cook the onion and juniper for 10 mins until the onion has softened, but not coloured.
2. Tip in the cabbage and fry for 10 mins, stirring, until it just starts to cook down.
3. Pour in the apple juice, season to taste, then cover and leave to simmer for 45 mins,

stirring occasionally, until the cabbage is tender and the liquid has almost all gone.

4. Add the cranberries, turn up the heat a little and continue to cook for about 5 mins until they have burst.

5. Check the seasoning and serve.

Turkey Meat Loaf With Walnuts And Sage

Ingredients:

- 2 tsp olive oil

- 1 large carrot, grated

- 4 scallions, thinly sliced

- 1 clove garlic, minced

- 1/2 cup walnuts (MUFA)

- 2 slices whole wheat bread

- 1/4 cup fat-free milk

- 2 egg whites, lightly beaten

- 1 pound extra-lean ground turkey breast (99% fat-free)

- 1/4 cup chopped fresh flat-leaf parsley

- 1/4 cup grated Parmesan cheese

- 1 tsp dried sage

- 1/2 tsp salt

- 1/2 tsp freshly ground black pepper

Directions:

1. Preheat the oven to 350°F. Line a rimmed baking sheet with foil and coat the foil with olive oil spray.

2. Heat the oil in a small nonstick skillet over medium heat.

3. Add the carrot, scallions, and garlic and cook, stirring often, for about 3 minutes or until tender. Remove from the heat.

4. Meanwhile, chop the walnuts in a food processor fitted with a metal blade.

5. Break up the bread and add to the walnuts. Pulse until both are ground to fine crumbs.

6. Transfer to a large bowl. With a fork, stir in the milk and egg whites.

7. Add the turkey, parsley, cheese, sage, salt, pepper, and sautéed mixture. Mix gently just until blended.

8. Shape into a free-form loaf about 7" long and 4 1/2" wide on the prepared baking sheet. Bake for 50 to 60 minutes or until a thermometer inserted in the thickest portion registers 165°F. Let stand a few minutes before slicing.

Slow Cooker Moroccan Chicken With Olives

Ingredients:

Chicken:

- 1/2 cup reduced-sodium chicken broth

- 1/4 cup all-purpose flour

- 3 Tbsp olive oil

- 2 tsp ground cumin

- 1/2 tsp freshly ground black pepper

- 1/4 tsp salt

- 1 can (14½ ounces) no-salt-added stewed tomatoes

- 1 carrot, sliced

- 1 large onion

- 30 small black olives, pitted (about 1 cup)

- 3 cloves garlic, minced

- 2 pounds boneless, skinless chicken breast halves

- 1/2 cup chopped fresh cilantro (optional)

Harissa:

- 3/4 cup dried hot red chile peppers, such as guajillo

- 2 cloves garlic, minced

- 1 tsp ground coriander

- 1 tsp ground caraway seed

- 1/4 tsp salt

- 3 Tbsp olive oil

Directions:

1. Prepare the chicken: Coat the stoneware of a slow cooker pot with cooking spray.

2. Combine the broth, flour, oil, cumin, pepper, and salt in the pot. Whisk until smooth.

3. Add the tomatoes (with juice), carrot, onion, olives, and garlic. Stir to mix.

4. Tuck the chicken into the pot, covering with the other INGREDIENTS:.

5. Cover and cook on low for 5 to 6 hours or on high for 3 to 4 hours.

6. Prepare the harissa: Remove the stems and seeds from the peppers and discard.

7. Soak the peppers in warm water for about 1 hour or until softened.

8. Drain and transfer to a food processor fitted with a metal blade or a blender.

9. Add the garlic, coriander, caraway seed, and salt.

10. Process, scraping the sides of the bowl as needed, until a paste forms.

11. Drizzle in the oil through the tube to reach a smooth consistency.

12. Stir in the cilantro (if using) just before serving. Pass the harissa at the table.

Quinoa Tabbouleh

Ingredients:

- 1 large English hothouse cucumber or 2 Persian cucumbers, cut into 1/4-inch pieces

- 1 pint cherry tomatoes, halved

- 2/3 cup chopped flat-leaf parsley

- 1/2 cup chopped fresh mint

- 2 scallions, thinly sliced

- 1 cup quinoa, rinsed well

- 1/2 tea spoon kosher salt plus more

- 2 table spoons fresh lemon juice

- 1 garlic clove, minced

- 1/2 cup extra-virgin olive oil

- Freshly ground black pepper

Directions:

1. Bring quinoa, 1/2 tsp. salt, and 1 1/4 cups water to a boil in a medium saucepan over high heat.

2. Reduce heat to medium-low, cover, and simmer until quinoa is tender, about 10 minutes.

3. Remove from heat and let stand, covered, for 5 minutes. Fluff with a fork.

4. Meanwhile, whisk lemon juice and garlic in a small bowl. Gradually whisk in olive oil. Season dressing to taste with salt and pepper.

5. Add cucumber, tomatoes, herbs, and scallions to bowl with quinoa; toss to coat.

6. Season to taste with salt and pepper. Drizzle remaining dressing over.

Beet And Arugula Salad With Quinoa, Avocado, And Sunflower Seeds

Ingredients:

- 2 ounces (¼ large) ounce avocado

- 1 ounce goat cheese

- 1 table spoon sunflower seeds

- ¼ cup leftover beets from Beet and Escarole Salad with Avocado and Walnuts

- 3 cups arugula

- ¼ cup quinoa

- Olive oil

- Lemon

Directions:

1. Toss beets with arugula, quinoa, olive oil, and lemon.

2. Top with avocado, goat cheese, and sunflower seeds.

Bananas Foster Vegan Ice Cream

Ingredients:

Ice cream:

- 1 cup unrefined sugar

- 2 tablespoons coconut oil

- 2 tablespoons coconut rum (optional)

- 3 ripe bananas smashed

- 2 cups almond or coconut milk alternative

- 8 oz plain Galaxy vegan cream cheese alternative, room temperature

- Unsweetened coconut flakes for garnish

Vegan caramel sauce:

- 2 tablespoons coconut oil

- 1 teaspoon vanilla extract

- 1/2 cup unrefined sugar

- 1/4 cup almond or coconut milk alternative

Directions:

Ice cream:

1. Place coconut oil and sugar in a sauce pan and cook over medium heat until sugar is melted, about 2 minutes.
2. Add the smashed bananas and vegan cream cheese.
3. Mix together and cook for another 3 minutes.
4. Mix in the coconut rum. Remove from heat and let the banana mixture cool for about 20 minutes.
5. Once cooled, combine the banana mixture and milk blend in a large bowl.
6. Mix well and pour the mixture into the ice cream maker.
7. Ice cream should be ready in about 20 minutes, depending on your ice cream maker.

Vegan caramel sauce:

1. Vegan Caramel Sauce:

2. Mix the sugar and milk in a sauce pan and bring to a boil over medium heat. Cook until mixture gets thick.

3. Remove from heat and mix in the coconut oil and vanilla extract.

Super Banana Oat Bars

Ingredients:

- 1/4 Cup Flour (your choice of flour; I ground more gluten-free oats in my spice grinder to a flour consistency)

- 1/2 Teaspoon Baking Soda

- 1/4 Teaspoon Salt

- 1 Egg (brought to room temperature if using coconut oil) or 1 Ener-G Egg Replacer

- 1 Cup Mashed, Ripe Banana (about 3 small or 2 large)

- 1-1/4 Cups Quick Oats (not instant)

- 1/4 Cup Honey or Agave Nectar

- 2 Tablespoons Coconut Oil, melted or softened (or baking oil of your choice)

- 1 Teaspoon Vanilla Extract

- 1/2 Cup Shredded Unsweetened Coconut

Directions:

1. Preheat your oven to 350ºF and grease an 8 x 8 baking dish.

2. In a medium mixing bowl, combine the oats, agave or honey, oil, and vanilla. Briefly set aside.

3. In a small bowl, combine the flour, baking soda, and salt. Briefly set aside.

4. Returning to your mixing bowl, stir in the egg, banana, and coconut, until everything is well combined.

5. Stir in the reserved flour mixture (since I was using oat flour without gluten, I wasn't worried about over-mixing.

6. Be careful not to over mix if you are using a wheat-based flour).

7. The batter will be a little thick.

8. Spread it evenly in your greased baking dish, and pop it in the oven for 25 to 30 minutes, or

until a toothpick inserted in the center comes
out clean.

9. Let cool completely before cutting. Can be
   stored in the fridge if you like them chilled (I
   do).

Potato Salad With Peas And Green Beans

Ingredients:

- 100g garden peas, fresh or frozen

- 100g watercress, washed

- 50g pea shoots (or baby spinach)

- 1 bunch radish, sliced in fine strips

- 1 tsp of fresh lemon juice, preferably extracted from ½ large-sized lemon

- 2 tbsp flax oil

- 500g baby new potatoes (or marble potatoes), sliced into halves

- 200g green beans, topped and tailed

- 5-8 pcs mint leaves, finely chopped

- Water

- Salt and pepper to season

Directions:

1. Put the halved potatoes in a saucepan with cold water, and bring to a boil. Let simmer for 10 minutes, or until potatoes are tender. Drain and place potatoes in a serving bowl, and season with salt and ground black pepper.

2. Boil another 2-3 cups of water to a boil, add the beans and let simmer for 90 seconds. Add the peas, and let simmer for another 90 seconds. Drain and add to the potatoes.

3. Add the watercress, pea shoots (or spinach), and radishes.

4. In a separate bowl, whisk the lemon juice, flax oil and finely chopped mint. Season with black pepper. Pour the mixture over the salad.

5. Toss and serve. This makes 2-3 servings.

Asparagus And Avocado Salad

Ingredients:

- ½ pc avocado, sliced

- 2 sprigs of asparagus

- 2 bunches or handfuls of mixed salad greens, fresh or frozen, sliced

- 1 pc tomato, sliced

- 1 pc cucumber, sliced

Directions:

1. In a bowl, place salad greens, tomato and cucumber. Mix lightly.
2. Top with avocado and asparagus. Toss, then serve.

Healthy Gourmet Goulash

Ingredients:

- 2 cups diced tomatoes (some utilization the canned variety)

- 2 carrots, chopped

- 2 zucchinis, chopped

- 1 onion (huge), chopped

- 2 15-ounce jars of your beloved beans (You can utilize kidney and garbanzo beans)

- 1 garlic clove, minced

- 1 cup elbow noodles (without gluten: rice noodles are my favorite)

- 1 pound ground hamburger (For a vegetarian rendition, you can exclude this by adding extra vegetables.)

- 1 teaspoon every one of paprika and oregano

71

- Salt and pepper

Directions:

1. Cook ground meat and the hacked onion in a skillet over medium hotness. While doing this, you can cook the elbow noodles as indicated by the guidelines on the package.
2. Mix the cooked noodles, beans, cleaved vegetables, and flavors in a major pan.
3. You can then add the onion and meat mixture.
4. Let everything stew on medium-low hotness for around 20 minutes or until the carrots become soft.
5. Enjoy your lunch!

Honey-Lime Chicken Skewers Key West Style

Ingredients:

- 1 tablespoon coconut oil

- 2 tablespoons honey

- Juice from one lime

- 1 to 2 teaspoons Siracha

- 2 minced garlic cloves

- 1 pound skinless and boneless chicken breasts

- 2 tablespoons cilantro

- 3 tablespoons soy sauce (check to ensure it is wheat-free)

- Red pepper drops, to taste

Directions:

1. In a little bowl, blend all fixings with the exception of the chicken.

2. Make certain to join everything thoroughly.

3. Pour the marinade over the chicken bosoms and go to cover them completely.

4. Cover and permit the marinade to absorb for no less than an hour.

5. Grill the chicken on medium high hotness for 6-8 minutes for each side. You will realize when it's done when the juices run clear.

Tropical Smoothie

Ingredients:

- 1 cup of strawberries

- 2-4cup of orange juice

- 6 ice cubes

- 2 mango (seeded)

- 2 papaya (cubed)

Directions:

1. Add mango, strawberries, and papaya in a blender. Blend the INGREDIENTS: until smooth.
2. Add ice cubes and orange juice for adjusting the consistency.
3. Blend again.
4. Serve with strawberry chunks from the top.

Fruit And Mint Smoothie

Ingredients:

- 2 tbsp. of lime juice

- 4 strawberries (frozen)

- 2 cup of pineapple cubes

- 4 mint leaves

- 2-4 cup of each

- Applesauce (unsweetened)

- Red grapes (seedless, frozen)

Directions:

1. Add grapes, lime juice, and applesauce in a blender. Blend the INGREDIENTS: until frothy and smooth.

2. Add pineapple cubes, mint leaves, and frozen strawberries in the blender.

3. Pulse the INGREDIENTS: for a few times until the pineapple and strawberries are crushed.

4. Serve with mint leaves from the top.

Good Old Steak And Eggs

Ingredients:

- Kosher salt, to taste

- 1/8 cup unsalted butter

- 6 large eggs

- 1 tablespoon peanut oil

- 1 lb. sirloin steak

Directions:

1. Preheat your oven to 350 degrees F.
2. Season the steak with salt and pepper.
3. Heat an oven proof skillet over medium high heat for 4-5 min.
4. Add the oil.
5. Pan fry the steak and flip every 203-0 sec. until browned on both sides. This takes about 3-4 min. per side.
6. Bake in the oven for 5-7 min.

Pork Chop Lunch Of The Week

Ingredients:

- ½ Cup Coconut Sugar

- ½ tsp Black Pepper

- ½ tsp Ginger

- 16-18 slices of Lean Pork Chops, around 4 ½ lbs.

- ¼ cup Light Soy Sauce

- 2/3 Cup Vinegar

Directions:

1. Preheat your oven to 350 degrees F.
2. Combine all of the INGREDIENTS: except the pork chop in a food processor to create the marinade.
3. Rub it all over the pork chops.
4. Bake for an hour and flip the pork chops at the 30 min. mark.

5. Slice into bite sized pieces.

6. Pack them into microwaveable containers

Spinach And Mushroom Egg Cups

Ingredients:

- 2 ½ cups liquid egg whites

- 3 large eggs, beaten well

- 2 tablespoons fat free milk

- 1 cup diced mushrooms

- 1 cup diced zucchini

- 1 cup frozen spinach, thawed and moisture squeezed out

- Fresh ground pepper

Directions:

1. Preheat the oven to 350°F and grease a muffin pan with cooking spray.

2. Combine the mushrooms, zucchini and spinach in a mixing bowl then spoon the mixture into the prepared muffin tin.

3. Beat together the egg whites, eggs, and milk then season with pepper.

4. Pour the egg mixture into the muffin cups, filling them almost to the top.

5. Bake for 20 to 30 minutes until the eggs are set and the tops browned.

Mixed Veggie Egg White Omelet

Ingredients:

- 1 clove minced garlic

- 3 large egg whites, beaten

- 1 tablespoon fresh chopped chives

- Pinch fresh ground pepper

- 2 teaspoons olive oil, divided

- ¼ cup fresh diced mushrooms

- ¼ cup fresh diced zucchini

- 2 tablespoons diced red pepper

Directions:

1. Heat 1 teaspoon oil in a small skillet over medium heat.

2. Add the mushrooms, red pepper, zucchini, and garlic then cook for 3 minutes.

3. Spoon the veggie mixture into a bowl and reheat the skillet with the rest of the oil.

4. Beat together the egg whites, chives and fresh pepper.

5. Pour the eggs into the skillet and cook for 1 minute then stir gently.

6. Cook the eggs for another 2 to 3 minutes until almost set.

7. Spoon the veggie mixture over half the omelet.

8. Fold the omelet over and cook for 1 minute or until the eggs are set.

Spinach Protein Smoothie

Ingredients:

- 1 scoop vanilla protein powder

- 1 tablespoon chia seeds

- 1 tablespoon flax meal

- ½ frozen banana

- ¼ cup frozen pineapple

- ¼ cup frozen mango chunks

- 1 handful of spinach, washed

Directions:

1. Combine the INGREDIENTS: in a blender and process until smooth.

Breakfast Smoothie

Ingredients:

- 4 oz. Vanilla Greek yogurt

- 1 orange, peeled and segmented

- 1 frozen banana

- 1 cup frozen mixed berries

Directions:

1. Combine all INGREDIENTS: in a blender and process until smooth.

Almond Butter Smoothie

Ingredients:

- 1 tablespoon chia seeds

- ¾ cup unsweetened almond milk

- 1 tablespoon unsweetened almond butter

- 1 ripe banana, peeled and frozen

Directions:

1. Mix the INGREDIENTS: in a blender and process until you get your desired consistency. Pour the smoothie into a glass and enjoy.

Coconut Chocolate Tart

Ingredients:

- Sweetener – should be equivalent to one cup of sugar

- 8 oz 100% chocolate

- 14 oz heavy cream or canned coconut milk

- 3 separated eggs

- 1/2 teaspoon vanilla extract

- 2 1/2 cups shredded coconut, unsweetened

- 2 teaspoons divided ground cinnamon

- 1/4 cup almond flour/meal

- 1/4 cup melted butter or coconut oil

Directions:

1. While preheating the oven to 350F, grease a 9-inch pie pan.

2. In a medium-sized bowl, combine your almond flour/meal, coconut, butter/oil, 1/4 cup sweetener and 1/2 tsp cinnamon and mix them thoroughly.
3. Transfer the mixture to your greased pie pan.
4. Spread it evenly on the bottom of the pie pan, and partially up the sides.
5. Bake this for 10 minutes, until the edges are lightly browned. Remove from the oven and allow to cool.
6. While your coconut shell is baking, heat your chocolate and cream or coconut milk over medium heat in a saucepan, until the chocolate melts.
7. Stir in your remaining sweetener.
8. Take care not to overheat the mixture. Remove it from heat.
9. Whip three egg whites until they form stiff peaks.

10. Reduce your speed and blend in the egg yolks, remaining cinnamon and vanilla.

11. Add your chocolate mixture with a spoon and blend it in with this mix gradually.

12. Pour your chocolate mixture into the coconut shell, and then bake for 15 additional minutes.

13. Remove from oven and allow to cool. Refrigerate until it sets. It is then ready to serve and enjoy.

Nutty Crunch Raisin Bars

Ingredients:

- 1 teaspoon vanilla extract

- 1 cup whey protein

- 1/2 cup almond butter, at room temperature

- 1/2 cup raisins, dried

- Sweetener that is equivalent to 1/2 cup of sugar

- 1/2 cup water

- 2 cups unsweetened coconut, shredded

- 2 teaspoons cinnamon, ground

- 1/4 cup melted coconut oil

- 1/2 cup walnut fragments

- 1/2 cup pumpkin seeds, raw

- 1/4 teaspoon sea salt

Directions:

1. Preheat your oven to 300F.

2. Combine cinnamon and coconut, and mix in a large bowl.

3. Mix vanilla and melted coconut oil in a smaller bowl. Add this to your coconut mixture. Mix this thoroughly and coat the coconut with oil.

4. Spread the mixture in a thin layer on a baking sheet. Bake for five minutes, then remove and toss lightly with a spoon. Continue to heat for an addition two or three minutes, until the mixture has browned lightly, and immediately remove. The idea is to remove the mixture as soon as it starts browning, or the coconut will burn.

5. Transfer the toasted coconut to the large bowl. Mix in pumpkin seeds, almond butter, water, salt, sweetener, whey protein, raisins and walnuts and combine.

6. Shape this mixture into bars and place on wax paper or parchment paper. Store them in the refrigerator.

7. Giving up wheat doesn't mean giving up tasty meals and snacks, especially since you won't be counting calories – just preparing foods without wheat.

Jewelled Cranberry & Juniper Red Cabbage

Ingredients:

- 1 large red cabbage , shredded

- 300ml good-quality apple juice

- 300g fresh or frozen cranberries

- 2 tbsp light olive oil

- 2 onions , halved and thinly sliced

- 1 tsp juniper berries, lightly crushed

Directions:

1. Heat the oil in a large lidded pan, then gently cook the onion and juniper for 10 mins until the onion has softened, but not coloured.

2. Tip in the cabbage and fry for 10 mins, stirring, until it just starts to cook down.

3. Pour in the apple juice, season to taste, then cover and leave to simmer for 45 mins,

stirring occasionally, until the cabbage is tender and the liquid has almost all gone.

4. Add the cranberries, turn up the heat a little and continue to cook for about 5 mins until they have burst.

5. Check the seasoning and serve.

Grilled Mediterranean Veg With Bean Mash

Ingredients:

- 1 red pepper , deseeded and quartered

- 1 aubergine , sliced lengthways

- 2 courgettes , sliced lengthways

- 2 tbsp olive oil

For the mash

- 100ml vegetable stock

- 1 tbsp chopped coriander

- lemon wedges, to serve

- 410g can haricot bean , rinsed

- 1 garlic clove , crushed

Directions:

1. Heat the grill. Arrange the vegetables over a grill pan and brush lightly with oil.

2. Grill until lightly browned, turn them over, brush again with oil, then grill until tender.

3. Meanwhile, put the beans in a small pan with the garlic and stock. Bring to the boil, then simmer, uncovered, for 10 mins.

4. Mash roughly with a potato masher, adding a little water or more stock if the mash seems too dry.

5. Divide the veg and mash between 2 plates, drizzle over any leftover oil and sprinkle with black pepper and coriander. Add a lemon wedge to each plate and serve.

Chicken Piccata

Ingredients:

- 12 ounces boneless, skinless chicken tenders

- 2 Tbsp flour

- 4 Tbsp olive oil

- 2 freshly squeezed lemon juice

- 2 Tbsp chopped fresh parsley

- 2 tsp capers, minced

- Freshly ground black pepper

Directions:

1. Lay the tenders on a work surface. With a smooth scaloppine pounder or a rolling pin covered in plastic wrap, flatten to 1/4" thickness.
2. Dredge the cutlets lightly in the flour.
3. Heat a large skillet over medium-high heat.

4. Add the oil to the skillet and heat until sizzling. Place the chicken in the skillet.

5. Cook for 2 minutes per side or until lightly browned and cooked through.

6. Add the lemon juice, parsley, and capers. Bring the mixture to a boil.

7. Reduce the heat and simmer for 2 minutes to allow the flavors to blend.

8. Season to taste with the pepper. Serve the chicken with the pan juices.

Slow Cooker African Chicken Stew

Ingredients:

- 1 Tbsp peanut oil

- 12 ounces boneless, skinless chicken thighs, trimmed and cut into 24 pieces

- 1 onion, chopped

- 3 cloves garlic, minced

- 1 jalapeno chile pepper, seeded and chopped

- 1 carrot, thickly sliced

- 1 sweet potato, peeled and cubed

- 1 can (14½ ounces) reduced-sodium chicken broth

- 1/2 cup chunky natural unsalted peanut butter

- 2 Tbsp tomato paste

- 1/4 tsp salt

100

- 1/4 tsp freshly ground black pepper

Directions:

1. Heat the oil in a large nonstick skillet over medium-high heat. Add the chicken and cook, stirring occasionally, for 3 to 4 minutes or until lightly browned.

2. Transfer to a 4-quart slow cooker. Return the skillet to the heat and add the onion, garlic, chile pepper, and carrot. Cook for 1 minute, then transfer to the slow cooker. Stir in the sweet potato, broth, peanut butter, and tomato paste.

3. Cook on high for 3 to 4 hours or low for 5 to 6 hours or until the chicken and vegetables are very tender. Season with salt and black pepper.

Red Quinoa With Parsley And Toasted Pine Nuts

Ingredients:

- Pinch of red pepper flakes, preferably Marash or Aleppo

- 1¼ cups red quinoa, rinsed

- ½ cup chopped fresh parsley

- ¼ cup toasted pine nuts

- 2 table spoons olive oil, plus more for drizzling

- 1 yellow onion, finely chopped

- Kosher salt

- ¾ tea spoon ground turmeric

Directions:

1. Heat oil in a medium saucepan over medium-high heat. Add onion and season with salt.

2. Cook, stirring often, until onion is tender and fragrant but not browned, about 4 minutes.

3. Reduce heat to medium and stir in turmeric and red pepper flakes. Cook until fragrant, about 30 seconds.

4. Add 1½ cups water and bring to a boil. Stir in quinoa and lower heat to a simmer.

5. Cover and cook until quinoa is tender and water is absorbed, 12–15 minutes.

6. Remove from heat. Let stand, covered, 10 minutes. Stir in parsley and pine nuts, and drizzle with oil.

Quinoa-Banana Muffins

Ingredients:

- Nonstick vegetable oil spray

- 1¼ cups whole wheat flour

- 1 tea spoon baking powder

- 1 tea spoon ground cinnamon

- 2 very ripe bananas

- ¼ cup honey

- ¼ cup (packed) dark brown sugar

- 1 large egg

- ½ cup olive oil

- ¾ cup white quinoa

- 1 tea spoon kosher salt, plus more

- 1 tea spoon vanilla extract

- 1 cup blueberries

- Raw sugar (for sprinkling)

Directions:

1. Cook quinoa in a large pot of boiling salted water, stirring occasionally, until tender, 10–12 minutes. Drain well and return to pot. Cover and let steam 10 minutes. Pour off any condensed water, then let cool. Set aside ¼ cup cooked quinoa for topping muffins.

2. Preheat oven to 375°. Coat a standard 12-cup muffin pan with nonstick spray (do not use muffin liners). Whisk flour, baking powder, cinnamon, and remaining 1 tsp. salt in a medium bowl.

3. Mash bananas, honey, and brown sugar in another medium bowl, preferably with a potato masher, until sugar is dissolved and banana is completely mashed. Add egg and continue to mash until combined. Stir in oil and vanilla.

4. Stir banana mixture into dry INGREDIENTS: just until combined. Stir in blueberries and 2 cups quinoa. Divide batter among muffin cups. Sprinkle lightly with raw sugar and reserved ¼ cup quinoa.

5. Bake muffins until tops are firm, just beginning to brown, and a tester inserted into muffins comes out clean, 30–40 minutes. Let cool slightly before serving.

Harissa-Roasted Broccoli, Tofu, And Quinoa Bowl

Ingredients:

- 2 table spoons harissa paste

- 7 table spoons olive oil, divided

- ¼ cup apple cider vinegar, divided

- Kosher salt, freshly ground pepper

- 1 large head of broccoli, cut into large florets with some stalk attached

- 1½ cups quinoa

- ½ pound extra-firm tofu

- 3 garlic cloves, grated

- ½ red onion, cut into ½-inch slices

- Sliced avocado and mint leaves (for serving)

Directions:

1. Real Talk: We're not trying to annoy you or put you through an unnecessary step by rinsing the quinoa, honest! Doing so removes the outer layer called saponin, which can lend an unpleasantly bitter flavor.

2. Preheat oven to 425°. Lay a clean kitchen towel or a double layer of paper towels on a large plate.

3. Place tofu on towel, then cover with another layer of towels. (Yes, it's a lot of towels.)

4. Cover with another plate and place something heavy (a few cans of beans or tomatoes will work) on plate to act as a weight.

5. Let sit at least 10 minutes; pressing out excess liquid in tofu is key to a crisp, not soggy, bowl. Remove weight and towels and cut tofu into ¾" pieces.

6. Whisk garlic, harissa, ¼ cup plus 2 Tbsp. oil, and 3 Tbsp. vinegar in a large bowl; generously season with salt and pepper. Toss broccoli and tofu in harissa mixture until coated.

7. Season with salt and pepper.

8. Transfer broccoli mixture to a rimmed baking sheet, spread out evenly, and roast, rotating sheet halfway through, until broccoli is lightly browned and cooked through, 30–40 minutes.

9. Meanwhile, place quinoa in a small bowl and cover with cold water. Let soak about 15 minutes, then drain through a fine-mesh sieve.

10. Cook quinoa in a large pot of boiling salted water, stirring occasionally so quinoa doesn't stick to bottom, until tender, 10–12 minutes.

11. Drain again; transfer to a medium bowl. Toss and fluff with remaining 1 Tbsp. oil and 1 Tbsp. vinegar; season with salt and pepper.

12. Divide quinoa among bowls. Top with broccoli mixture, onion, avocado, and mint.

Homemade Fruit-Sweetened Oat Milk

Ingredients:

- pinch of salt (optional)

- 1 teaspoon vanilla extract (optional)

- Sweetener to taste (optional)

- 4 to 5 cups cold water

- 1 ripe banana

- 2 cups raw or cooked oatmeal

Directions:

1. Place all INGREDIENTS: in a blender and process for 2 to 3 minutes.
2. Strain through a fine mesh strainer or cheesecloth.

3. Chill the oat milk in the refrigerator until ready to use.
4. It may thicken further. If so, you can thin with additional water.

Low Calorie Dairy-Free Eggnog

Ingredients:

- 1-3+ tablespoons no sugar maple syrup (sweeten to taste)

- 1/2 teaspoon cinnamon (or more to taste)

- 1/2 teaspoon nutmeg (or more to taste)

- 2 cups vanilla soy milk such as ZenSoy Organic Soymilk

- 1 egg

Directions:

1. Blend well
2. Heat slowly until 180ºF, but stop before a boil.
3. Cool or drink warm.

Creamy Cauliflower Salad

Ingredients:

- 5 tbsp mayonnaise, low-fat option

- 2 tbsp cider vinegar

- 1 pc shallot, finely chopped

- ¼ tsp ground pepper

- 3 cups cauliflower florets, chopped

- 2 cups romaine, heart part, chopped

- 1 pc red apple, chopped

Directions:

1. In a large bowl, whisk mayonnaise, vinegar, shallot, and ground pepper, until smooth.
2. Add in cauliflower florets, romaine, and apple slices. Toss. This makes 5-6 servings.

Vegetable Stir-Fry

Ingredients:

- ½ tray sugar snap peas

- 1 pc small ginger, chopped

- ½ clove garlic, crushed

- 1 tsp coconut butter

- ¾ tsp Tamari sauce

- ½ head broccoli, chopped

- ½ pc fennel, sliced

- 1 pc courgette, sliced

- Some coriander, chopped

Directions:

1. Fry ginger and garlic on coconut butter until lightly brown.
2. Add broccoli, fennel, courgette and sugar snap peas.

3. Add Tamari sauce and a little water. Fry while stirring and letting the vegetable steam through.
4. Remove from fire, top with chopped coriander as garnishing.
5. Serve with rice. This makes 3-4 servings.

Mushroom Risotto

Ingredients:

- 7 ounces risotto rice (Arborio)

- 1 onion, chopped

- 1 green pepper, chopped

- 1 red pepper, chopped

- 2 tablespoons olive oil

- 7 ounces grams grouped mushrooms, sliced

- 750 ml sans wheat or sans gluten vegetable stock

- 2 teaspoons dried oregano

- ounces of parmesan cheddar, ground (for vegetarian adaptation, discard this or use sans dairy parmesan)

- Additional bubbling water

- Freshly ground dark pepper

Directions:

1. In a weighty lined skillet, put 2 tablespoon olive oil or coconut oil and add the rice.

2. Delicately heat the rice for around 2-3 minutes, until the rice looks translucent.

3. Add the onion, mushrooms, and peppers, and cook for an additional 5 minutes.

4. Be mindful so as not to brown the rice.

5. Add vegetable stock and heat to the point of boiling.

6. Lessen the hotness and stew the rice for around 25 minutes.

7. Add bubbling water as important, to ensure that the combination doesn't dry out.

8. When cooking is done, the risotto ought to be soggy, delicate, and rich, not dry. It is smarter to leave the risotto somewhat wetter than concoct a dry one.

9. Add the oregano and dark pepper. Blend well.

10. Serve with ground parmesan on top, or for a vegetarian rendition, with sans dairy armesan.

Banana Smoothie

Ingredients:

- 2 tbsp. of honey

- 9 cubes of ice

- 4 bananas (sliced)

- 2 cup of fresh pineapple juice

Directions:

1. Combine the bananas and pineapple juice in a blender.
2. Blend until smooth.
3. Add ice cubes along with honey.
4. Blend for two minutes.
5. Serve immediately.

Dragon Fruit Smoothie

Ingredients:

- 2 cup of yogurt

- 2 dragon fruit (chopped)

- 2 cup of pineapple cubes

- 2 tbsp. of honey

- 1-3 cup of almonds

- 2 tbsps. of shredded coconut

- 1e tsp. of chocolate chips

Directions:

1. Add almonds, dragon fruit, coconut, and chocolate chips in a high power blender. Blend until smooth.
2. Add yogurt, pineapple, and honey. Blend well.
3. Serve with chunks of dragon fruit from the top.

Taco Salad

Ingredients:

- 6 Romaine Lettuce Leafs

- 6 tsp. Taco Seasoning

- Chili Powder, to taste

- 32 oz Ground Pork

- 9 oz. Monterey Jack Cheese, shredded

- 2 cups Salsa

Directions:

1. Heat the oil in a pan over medium high heat.
2. Stir fry the ground pork until browned.
3. Add the taco seasoning and chili powder.
4. Divide the ground pork mixture among 5-6 containers.
5. Divide the rest of the INGREDIENTS: on the containers.

Mason Jar Salad

Ingredients:

- 2 Tbsp Extra Virgin Olive Oil

- 2 Tbsp Mayonnaise

- 1 Tbsp Lemon Juice

- 1 tsp Distilled White Vinegar

- 1 Tbsp Dill

- 1 tsp Parsley

- Lbs Asparagus Spears, ends trimmed off and cut into 1 inch bite sized pieces

- 9 Radishes, thinly sliced

- 3 Oz Sour Cream

- Pepper to taste

Directions:

1. Boil some salted water and add the asparagus until it turns bright green and place in a bowl of cold water.

2. Combine the rest of the INGREDIENTS: except the radish in a food processor.

3. Toss the INGREDIENTS: together and place them in mason jars

Avocado Walnut Smoothie

Ingredients:

- 2 tablespoons chopped walnuts

- 1 cup skim milk

- 1 tablespoon fresh lime juice

- 1 small frozen banana, peeled and chopped

- ½ cup fresh chopped avocado

- 1 small stalk celery, sliced

Directions:

1. Combine all of the INGREDIENTS: in a high-speed blender.
2. Blend for 30 to 60 seconds on high speed until smooth.
3. Pour the smoothie into a glass and enjoy immediately.

Carrot And Ginger Soup

Ingredients:

- 1 tablespoon fresh minced ginger

- 1 tablespoon fresh minced garlic

- 6 cups vegetable broth

- 1 tablespoon olive oil

- 1 ½ lbs. carrots, peeled and sliced

- 2 medium Yukon gold potatoes, peeled and chopped

Directions:

1. Heat the oil in a large saucepan over medium-high heat.

2. Add the carrots, potato, ginger and garlic and cook for 5 minutes.

3. Stir in the broth and bring the mixture to a boil.

4. Reduce heat and simmer for 25 to 30 minutes until the vegetables are tender.

5. Remove from heat and puree the soup using an immersion blender. Serve hot.

Yummy Miniature Pizzas

Ingredients:

- 1/2 cup ground flaxseed

- 1 teaspoon sea salt

- 2 tablespoons olive oil

- 1 1/2 cups sugar-free marinara or pizza sauce

- 3/4 cup of warm water

- 1 1/4 teaspoons active dry yeast

- 1 cup almond flour/meal

- 1 cup chickpea flour

Toppings are optional:

- 1 cup mozzarella cheese – shredded

- 1 cup ricotta cheese

- 4 oz thin-sliced pepperoni

- 8 oz thin sliced mozzarella cheese – fresh

- Thin sliced, sautéed onion and bell pepper

- Thin sliced, sautéed zucchini and yellow squash

- Grape tomatoes – quartered

- 2 tablespoons fresh, chopped herbs

Directions:

1. Whisk the yeast and water in a small sized bowl until the yeast fully dissolves.
2. Allow this to stand for 10 minutes.
3. Whisk the almond flour/meal, chickpea flour, salt and flaxseed in a medium bowl.
4. Add the yeast and oil mixture and stir together for five minutes, until all of your INGREDIENTS: are distributed evenly and formed into a ball of dough.
5. Cover the dough ball with plastic wrap and allow it to stand in a warm area for one hour. Then divide the ball into six equal pieces.

6. Preheat your oven to 350F. Line two baking sheets with parchment paper.

7. Use a piece of the same type of parchment paper on your work surface. Place one dough piece on parchment paper and top it with a second parchment paper sheet. Flatten it into a four-inch circle with a rolling pin.

8. Place your dough circle on a baking sheet. Remove the top parchment paper carefully. Use your hands or a spoon to form the crust edge. Repeat these steps with the other dough pieces.

9. Bake the dough pieces for 20 minutes, or until they are lightly brown. Then remove them from the oven and top them with 1/4 cup marinara or pizza sauce and your favorite toppings. Bake for 10 more minutes or until they are heated all the way through.

Honey-Roasted Swede With Chilli & Cumin

Ingredients:

- 1 tsp cumin seed

- 1 large red chilli , deseeded and chopped

- small bunch coriander , chopped

- 1 large swede , peeled and cut into large chunks

- 2 tbsp olive oil

- 1 tbsp clear honey

Directions:

1. Heat oven to 200C/180C fan/gas 6. Toss the swede in olive oil in a shallow roasting tin, then season.

2. Roast in the oven for 35-40 mins, tossing occasionally, until the swede is golden and soft.

3. Stir in the honey and cumin seeds, and continue to roast for 10 mins until just starting to catch.

4. Remove and stir through the chilli and coriander to serve.

Mediterranean Fish Stew With Garlic Toasts

Ingredients:

- 1 red chilli , finely chopped

- 2 tbsp tomato purée

- 1kg tomatoes , roughly chopped

- 200ml white wine

- 350ml fish stock

- 3 strips orange zest

- 1kg skinless halibut fillets, cut into large chunks

- 500g clams

- 3 tbsp olive oil

- 1 large onion , sliced

- 2 garlic cloves , sliced

- 400g large raw prawns

132

- Handful flat-leaf parsley , chopped

- For the garlic toasts

- 1 large ciabatta loaf, cut into 1cm slices

- 5 tbsp olive oil

- 2 garlic cloves , halved

Directions:

1. To make the garlic toasts, drizzle the bread with oil, then griddle or grill until golden all over. While the toasts are still hot, rub them with garlic and set aside.

2. Heat the oil in a wide, deep frying pan. Add the onion and cook over a gentle heat for 5 mins until softened. Stir through the garlic and chilli and cook a couple of mins more. Add the tomato purée and tomatoes. Turn up the heat and cook for 10-15 mins, stirring until the tomatoes are pulpy. Pour over the wine

and cook for 10 mins more until most of it has boiled away.

3. Add the fish stock and orange zest and heat until gently simmering. Nestle the halibut chunks into the liquid and cook for 5 mins. Add the clams and prawns and cook for 5 mins more until the fish is cooked through and the clams have opened (discard any that haven't). Sprinkle the parsley over the stew and serve with the garlic toasts.

Spicy Olive And Turkey Pita Sandwich

Ingredients:

- 10 pitted green pimiento-stuffed olives,chopped

- 10 pitted black olives, chopped

- 1 tsp balsamic vinegar

- 1 tsp extra virgin olive oil

- 1/8 tsp red-pepper flakes

- 1 whole wheat (6" diameter) pita, halved crosswise

- 4 ounces deli-sliced lower-sodium turkey breast

- 1/2 cup mixed greens

Directions:

1. Combine the green and black olives, vinegar, oil, and red-pepper flakes in a small bowl.

2. Fill each pita half with 2 ounces turkey breast, 1/4 cup greens, and half of the olive mixture.

Escarole Salad With Anchovy Cream And Crispy Quinoa

Ingredients:

- 2 tea spoons apple cider vinegar

- 2 tea spoons Dijon mustard

- ½ tea spoon honey

- 6 cups torn escarole (from about 2 small heads)

- ½ cup mixed herb leaves (such as parsley and/or dill)

- Freshly ground black pepper

- ¼ cup red or white quinoa

- Kosher salt

- Vegetable oil (for frying; about 1 cup)

- 6 oil-packed anchovy fillets, chopped

- 1 garlic clove, chopped

- ⅓ cup heavy cream

- Shaved Parmesan (for serving)

Directions:

1. Cook quinoa in a small pot of boiling salted water until tender, 10–15 minutes. Drain and transfer to a paper towel–lined rimmed baked sheet. Let sit, tossing occasionally, until dry, 20–25 minutes.

2. Pour oil to come ¼" up the sides of a medium skillet; heat over medium-high. Fry quinoa, stirring occasionally, until sizzling subsides, about 3 minutes. Transfer to paper towels to drain.

3. Place anchovies, garlic, and a pinch of salt on a cutting board. Using the side of a chef's knife, smash anchovies and garlic into a paste (this can also be done in a mortar and pestle).

Transfer paste to a medium bowl and whisk in cream, vinegar, mustard, and honey.

4. Add escarole and herbs to anchovy cream; season with salt and pepper and toss to combine.

5. Serve salad topped with fried quinoa and Parmesan.

6. Do Ahead: Quinoa can be fried 1 day ahead; store airtight at room temperature. Anchovy cream can be made 1 day ahead; cover and chill.